You & BABY™
Pregnancy
ORGANIZER

Copyright © 2006 by Meredith Corporation.

All rights reserved. No part of this book may be reproduced in any form without written permission from the publisher.

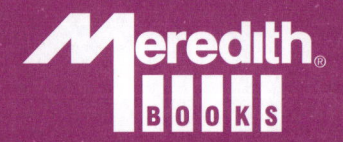

Meredith® BOOKS

Meredith Books
1716 Locust Street
Des Moines, Iowa 50309–3023
www.meredithbooks.com

First Edition. Printed in China.
Library of Congress Control Number: 2005929471
ISBN: 0-696-22829-7

You and Your Baby is a trademark of Meredith Corporation.

Congratulations Mom-to-Be!

Your pregnancy promises to be one of the most exciting times in your life. Although you are positive that you'll remember every little detail of this journey—from the first time you felt your baby hiccup to your first outing in maternity jeans—it's likely that your memories will fade as the days and months pass. Someday you may want to write those details in the pretty baby books you'll get at your baby showers, and this log will help jog your memory. There are excellent medical reasons for tracking your progress too: in case you need to switch prenatal providers during pregnancy, in the event that your insurance company asks for information, and to check that you're on track with the diet, exercise, and medication recommendations your provider makes. Stash this book in your purse or your car so it's always close by.

Contents

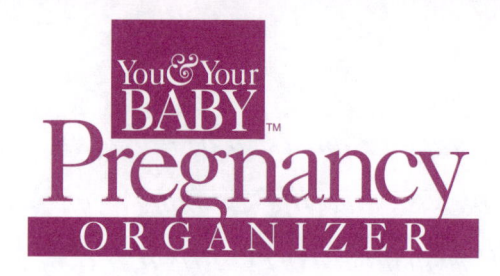

You & Your BABY™ Pregnancy ORGANIZER

SECTION 1: Oh, Baby! My Prenatal Care 7
   My Due Date 8
   How to Use "My Pregnancy Calendar" 9
   My Pregnancy Calendar 10
   I'm Pregnant, World! 30
   Choosing My Doctor 31
   My Doctor 35
   My Medical History 36
   My Partner's and Family Medical History 40
   Good Question! 42
   Testing, Testing 44
   My Prenatal Visits 52
   Monitoring My Baby's Movements 76
   Finding a Pediatrician 80
   My Firsts 83

SECTION 2: Eat, Drink (Water), and Be Merry 85
   My Food and Diet Progress 86
   My Food Cravings 128

SECTION 3: At Work and at Home **131**
    Evaluating Home Hazards 132
    Evaluating Work Hazards 136
    Maternity Leave 140
    Final Checklist for Leaving Work 145

SECTION 4: And Baby Makes Three (or More!) **147**
    Go to the Head of the Class 148
    Retail Therapy 150
    Off to the Hospital 158
    Words of Wisdom 164
    It's Delivery Day! 166
    My Labor (Finally!) 168
    My Contractions 174
    My Labor and Delivery 177
    My Partner's Labor Experience 178
    My Labor Team 180
    Baby's First Visitors 182
    What a Surprise! 184

SECTION 5: It's a Celebration! **185**
    Baby Showers 186
    Baby Announcements 192
    Name Games 200
    Phone or E-mail Tree 204
    Handy Websites 207

How to Use this Book

If you have a pen or pencil in your hand, then you're ready to make good use of the You & Your Baby: Pregnancy Organizer. *Don't think of this as a traditional book that you read from front to back. Instead think of it as a prenatal workbook, notebook, to-do list, and baby organizer all wrapped into one. Although the book is divided into five sections, you'll probably find yourself using pages from each section at the same time. So take a few minutes to flip through the book.*

This is meant to be a workbook where you can scribble important reminders (like the adorable baby name you just heard) and make notes during your visits to the doctor. Don't worry about whether or not your handwriting is pretty; if you have important memories you'd like to keep, you can transfer them to a scrapbook or baby book later.

Oh, Baby!
My Prenatal Care

1

My Due Date	.8
How to Use "My Pregnancy Calendar"	.9
My Pregnancy Calendar	.10
I'm Pregnant, World!	.30
Choosing My Doctor	.31
My Doctor	.35
My Medical History	.36
My Partner's and Family Medical History	.40
Good Question!	.42
Testing, Testing	.44
My Prenatal Visits	.52
Monitoring My Baby's Movements	.76
Finding a Pediatrician	.80
My Firsts	.83

Oh, Baby!
My Prenatal Care

1

You'll likely see your prenatal provider more in the next 9 months than you've seen your regular doctor in the past 9 years. Make the most of your visits by jotting down lists of your questions, noting your test results, and keeping logs of vitamins and medications you may be taking. This is a critical time in your baby's development, even though it will still be months before you hear your baby cry for the first time. By getting good prenatal care, you'll give your baby the healthiest possible start to his (or her!) exciting new life.

My Due Date

One question near the top of your list is likely this: When is my baby due? Your doctor will calculate your official due date at your first prenatal exam, which is usually scheduled during week 9 or 10 of your pregnancy. Can't wait until then? Make your own estimate.

How to calculate your due date:

1. Grab a calendar.

2. Write down the first day of your last normal menstrual period (March 17, for example).

3. Add exactly 9 months and 7 days to that date to get your due date (December 24, for example).

My last normal menstrual period started on: _____

_____

Adding 9 months and 7 days comes to this date: _____

_____

motherly ADVICE **Only 5 percent of babies** are actually born on their estimated due dates. Be prepared for your baby to arrive sooner—or later!

How to Use "My Pregnancy Calendar"

Your pregnancy is measured in weeks, and it'll be about 40 weeks until you meet your sweet baby. Fill in these calendars to remind yourself of key events or appointments and to track your progress toward your due date. (See the sample below.) Include scheduled visits with your prenatal provider, midwife, doula, daycare providers, or if you like, your hairdresser.

Month: **January 2007**

Week of my pregnancy	SUNDAY	MONDAY	TUESDAY	WEDNESDAY	THURSDAY	FRIDAY	SATURDAY
9		1	2	3	4 9 a.m. Dentist appointment	5	6
10	7	8 Pick up prenatal vitamins	9	10	11	12	13
11	14	15	16	17 2 p.m. Doctor's visit	18	19	20
12	21	22	23	24	25	26 10 a.m. Meeting at daycare	27
13	28	29	30	31			

9

My Pregnancy Calendar

Month: _____

Week of my pregnancy:	SUNDAY	MONDAY	TUESDAY
_____			
_____			
_____			
_____			
_____			

WEDNESDAY	THURSDAY	FRIDAY	SATURDAY

My Pregnancy Calendar

Month: _____

Week of my pregnancy:	SUNDAY	MONDAY	TUESDAY
_____			
_____			
_____			
_____			
_____			

WEDNESDAY	THURSDAY	FRIDAY	SATURDAY

My Pregnancy Calendar

Month: _____

Week of my pregnancy:	SUNDAY	MONDAY	TUESDAY
_____			
_____			
_____			
_____			
_____			

WEDNESDAY	THURSDAY	FRIDAY	SATURDAY

My Pregnancy Calendar

Month:_____

Week of my pregnancy:	SUNDAY	MONDAY	TUESDAY

WEDNESDAY	THURSDAY	FRIDAY	SATURDAY

My Pregnancy Calendar

Month:_____

Week of my pregnancy:	SUNDAY	MONDAY	TUESDAY
_____			
_____			
_____			
_____			
_____			

WEDNESDAY	THURSDAY	FRIDAY	SATURDAY

My Pregnancy Calendar

Month: _____

Week of my pregnancy:	SUNDAY	MONDAY	TUESDAY
_____			
_____			
_____			
_____			
_____			

WEDNESDAY	THURSDAY	FRIDAY	SATURDAY

My Pregnancy Calendar

Month: _____

Week of my pregnancy:	SUNDAY	MONDAY	TUESDAY
_____			
_____			
_____			
_____			
_____			

WEDNESDAY	THURSDAY	FRIDAY	SATURDAY

My Pregnancy Calendar

Month: _____

Week of my pregnancy:	SUNDAY	MONDAY	TUESDAY
_____			
_____			
_____			
_____			
_____			

WEDNESDAY	THURSDAY	FRIDAY	SATURDAY

My Pregnancy Calendar

Month: _____

Week of my pregnancy:	SUNDAY	MONDAY	TUESDAY
_____			
_____			
_____			
_____			
_____			

WEDNESDAY	THURSDAY	FRIDAY	SATURDAY

My Pregnancy Calendar

Month: _____

Week of my pregnancy:	SUNDAY	MONDAY	TUESDAY
_____			
_____			
_____			
_____			
_____			

WEDNESDAY	THURSDAY	FRIDAY	SATURDAY

I'm Pregnant, World!

The date I suspected I might be pregnant:

_____

_____

What made me suspicious:

_____

_____

_____

The date I confirmed my pregnancy:

_____

_____

_____

How I told my partner the news:

_____

_____

_____

What my other children said when I told them:

_____

_____

_____

The date I shared the news with my family and friends:

_____

_____

_____

Choosing My Doctor

Who will deliver your baby? When interviewing doctors and choosing a hospital or birth center, ask lots of questions and take notes. If you already have a doctor, look over the following questions to see whether you've already discussed them with your doctor.

Interview #1

Doctor's Name:

Hospital or birth center:

Address:

Phone number:

SUGGESTED QUESTIONS:

Where do you deliver? Is it at a hospital? A birth center?

What prenatal tests do you suggest?

Who will deliver my baby if you're not around?

Choosing My Doctor

When do you recommend a cesarean delivery?

What's your philosophy on pain management during labor?

What's your philosophy on episiotomies?

What's your philosophy on circumcision?

Can I call you between appointments?

Other questions:

Interview #2

Doctor's Name: _____

Hospital or birth center: _____

_____

Address: _____

_____

_____

Phone number: _____

_____

SUGGESTED QUESTIONS:

Where do you deliver? Is it at a hospital? A birth center?

_____

_____

_____

What prenatal tests do you suggest?

_____

_____

_____

Who will deliver my baby if you're not around?

_____

_____

_____

When do you recommend a cesarean delivery?

What's your philosophy on pain management during labor?

What's your philosophy on episiotomies?

What's your philosophy on circumcision?

Can I call you between appointments?

Other questions:

My Doctor

NAME: _____
_____

Address: _____
_____
_____

Office phone number: _____

After-hours phone number: _____

Office hours: _____
_____
_____

My insurance information: _____
_____
_____
_____
_____
_____
_____

doctor's ADVICE

How often will your prenatal provider schedule regular checkups? If your pregnancy is without complications, your visits will likely follow this schedule:

Weeks 4 to 28: One visit every 4 weeks
Weeks 28 to 36: Two visits every month
Weeks 36 to birth: One visit every week

My Medical History

Be prepared to share detailed information on your health history—and that of your partner and family—at your first prenatal visit. The more specific you are, the better able your provider will be to care for you and your baby.

Chronic illnesses I have:

Medications I'm taking (including how often they're taken, dosages, and reasons for use):

Allergies:

Surgeries:

Start date of last menstrual period: _____
_____
_____

Date of last Pap smear: _____
_____
_____

Fertility issues, if any: _____
_____
_____
_____
_____

Fertility treatments, if any: _____
_____
_____
_____

Number of previous pregnancies: _____
_____
_____

doctor's ADVICE

Instead of writing down the details of all your prescriptions, take the prescription containers with you to your first appointment—along with any over-the-counter (OTC) vitamins or herbal supplements you're taking—so that you can talk to your doctor about safe medication use during pregnancy.

My Medical History

Complications during previous pregnancies and deliveries:
_____
_____
_____
_____

Number of miscarriages (include the dates):
_____
_____
_____
_____

Number of abortions, if any (include the dates):
_____
_____
_____
_____

Are you a smoker? Yes/No   How often?
_____
_____

> **doctor's ADVICE**
>
> **Prenatal vitamins are available** over-the-counter (OTC) at your local drugstore or by prescription. OTC vitamins are perfectly safe to take, as long as they are labeled as "prenatal vitamins." It's wise to start taking prenatal vitamins right now, especially if your first doctor's visit is still several weeks away.

Do you drink alcohol? Yes/No　　How often?

Have you ever used or are you using street drugs?

Do you have any sexually transmitted diseases?

Type:

Other important notes:

My Partner's and Family Medical History

Some health problems are more likely to occur in certain families, racial groups, or ethnic groups. In order to assess your baby's risk of developing or inheriting diseases, your doctor will ask you about your partner's health history as well as your family history. Check any conditions that apply.

	You	Your partner	Your other children, if any
Alcohol abuse			
Allergies:			
Peanut allergy			
Others _____ (such as soy, dairy, seafood, or wheat)			
Asthma			
Cancer			
Cystic fibrosis			
Diabetes			
Down syndrome			
Drug abuse			
Heart disease (high cholesterol, high blood pressure)			
Mental retardation			
Obesity			
Sexually transmitted diseases			
Sickle-cell anemia			
Spina bifida			
Tay-Sachs disease			
Others _____			

Your parents	Your partner's parents	Your grandparents	Your partner's grandparents
_____	_____	_____	_____
_____	_____	_____	_____
_____	_____	_____	_____
_____	_____	_____	_____
_____	_____	_____	_____
_____	_____	_____	_____
_____	_____	_____	_____
_____	_____	_____	_____
_____	_____	_____	_____
_____	_____	_____	_____
_____	_____	_____	_____
_____	_____	_____	_____
_____	_____	_____	_____

Good Question!

Prepare for your first prenatal visit by writing down any questions you may have for your doctor. Use this list to get yourself started.

- What type of bleeding is normal—and what is not normal?
- How many ultrasounds will I have and when?
- What are the benefits and drawbacks of prenatal screenings?
- Is it safe for me to travel by car? By plane?
- How long can I continue to work?
- What exercises are recommended during pregnancy?
- Is it OK to continue to color my hair?
- How much weight should I gain?
- If I weigh more than I should, can I cut back on my meals?
- When is the best time to start childbirth classes?
- What can I do to relieve my heartburn?
- Can I get a pregnancy massage?
- If my baby seems quiet or does not move, what should I do?
- Can my partner videotape the delivery?
- If my mom had a cesarean delivery, will I have one also?
- Is it normal for my feet to swell?
- If I do not deliver by my due date, what happens?
- Is it all right if I bring my partner or friend to prenatal visits?

My questions

Answers

Testing, Testing

Keep track of your medical results with this list of the most common prenatal tests. Use the "other tests" section (pages 48-51) to record any additional tests you may undergo.

TEST: Blood type
Purpose: Determines whether your blood type is A, B, AB, or O. This information must be in your medical record in case you need a blood transfusion.

Date: _____

Results: _____

Notes: _____

_____

_____

_____

_____

TEST: Rh factor
Purpose: Determines whether your blood is Rh-negative or Rh-positive. If you are Rh-negative and your partner is Rh-positive (his blood may be tested too), your pregnancy will require closer monitoring.

Date: _____

Results: _____

Notes: _____

_____

_____

_____

_____

TEST: Hemoglobin/hematocrit
Purpose: Indicates vitamin B₁₂, folate, and iron deficiency. If you're low in iron, you may need an iron supplement in addition to the iron you get in your prenatal vitamin.

Date: _____

Results: _____

Notes: _____

_____

_____

_____

_____

_____

_____

TEST: Hepatitis B
Purpose: Detects this viral infection of the liver. Left untreated, hepatitis B can cause life-threatening liver diseases. Treatment can prevent the virus from passing to your baby.

Date: _____

Results: _____

Notes: _____

_____

_____

_____

_____

_____

Testing, Testing

TEST: **Urine culture**
Purpose: Checks for the presence of bacteria. Bacteria in the urine, if not treated with antibiotics, may lead to a kidney infection.

Date:

Results:

Notes:

TEST: **Pap**
Purpose: Checks for cancerous or precancerous cells in the cervix.

Date:

Results:

Notes:

TEST: CVS (chorionic villus sampling)
Purpose: Tests for Down syndrome, Tay-Sachs disease, and 200 other disorders.

Date:

Results:

Notes:

TEST: Multiple marker screening test (also known as a quad screen)
Purpose: Detects chromosomal abnormalities such as Down syndrome and neural tube defects.

Date:

Results:

Notes:

Testing, Testing

TEST: Amniocentesis (also called an "amnio")
Purpose: Can detect Down syndrome and other chromosomal disorders, including Tay-Sachs disease, cystic fibrosis, and sickle-cell anemia.

Date:

Results:

Notes:

Other tests

TEST:

Purpose:

Date:

Results:

Notes:

TEST:

Purpose:

Date:

Results:

Notes:

TEST:

Purpose:

Date:

Results:

Notes:

Testing, Testing

TEST:

Purpose:

Date:

Results:

Notes:

TEST:

Purpose:

Date:

Results:

Notes:

TEST:

Purpose:

Date:

Results:

Notes:

TEST:

Purpose:

Date:

Results:

Notes:

My Prenatal Visits

Visit #1

Prenatal provider seen:

Date:

The week of my pregnancy:

Weight:

Weight gain since the start of my pregnancy:

Blood pressure:

Fundal height:

Baby's heart rate:

Other tests:

Prescribed medications:

_____
_____
_____

What I can expect before my next prenatal visit:

_____
_____
_____

Instructions from my doctor:

_____
_____
_____

How much weight I should gain:

_____
_____
_____

Notes:

_____
_____
_____
_____
_____

My Prenatal Visits

Visit #2

Prenatal provider seen:

Date:

The week of my pregnancy:

Weight:

Weight gain since the start of my pregnancy:

Blood pressure:

Fundal height:

Baby's heart rate:

Other tests:

Prescribed medications:

What I can expect before my next prenatal visit:

Instructions from my doctor:

How much weight I should gain:

Notes:

My Prenatal Visits

Visit #3

Prenatal provider seen:

Date:

The week of my pregnancy:

Weight:

Weight gain since the start of my pregnancy:

Blood pressure:

Fundal height:

Baby's heart rate:

Other tests:

Prescribed medications:

What I can expect before my next prenatal visit:

Instructions from my doctor:

How much weight I should gain:

Notes:

My Prenatal Visits

Visit #4

Prenatal provider seen:

Date:

The week of my pregnancy:

Weight:

Weight gain since the start of my pregnancy:

Blood pressure:

Fundal height:

Baby's heart rate:

Other tests:

Prescribed medications:

_____
_____
_____
_____

What I can expect before my next prenatal visit:

_____
_____
_____
_____

Instructions from my doctor:

_____
_____
_____
_____

How much weight I should gain:

_____
_____
_____
_____

Notes:

_____
_____
_____
_____
_____
_____

My Prenatal Visits

Visit #5

Prenatal provider seen:

Date:

The week of my pregnancy:

Weight:

Weight gain since the start of my pregnancy:

Blood pressure:

Fundal height:

Baby's heart rate:

Other tests:

Prescribed medications:

What I can expect before my next prenatal visit:

Instructions from my doctor:

How much weight I should gain:

Notes:

My Prenatal Visits

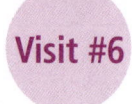

Visit #6

Prenatal provider seen:

Date:

The week of my pregnancy:

Weight:

Weight gain since the start of my pregnancy:

Blood pressure:

Fundal height:

Baby's heart rate:

Other tests:

Prescribed medications:

What I can expect before my next prenatal visit:

Instructions from my doctor:

How much weight I should gain:

Notes:

My Prenatal Visits

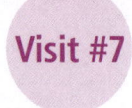

Visit #7

Prenatal provider seen:

Date:

The week of my pregnancy:

Weight:

Weight gain since the start of my pregnancy:

Blood pressure:

Fundal height:

Baby's heart rate:

Other tests:

Prescribed medications:
_____
_____
_____
_____

What I can expect before my next prenatal visit:
_____
_____
_____
_____

Instructions from my doctor:
_____
_____
_____
_____

How much weight I should gain:
_____
_____
_____
_____

Notes:
_____
_____
_____
_____
_____
_____

My Prenatal Visits

Visit #8

Prenatal provider seen:

Date:

The week of my pregnancy:

Weight:

Weight gain since the start of my pregnancy:

Blood pressure:

Fundal height:

Baby's heart rate:

Other tests:

Prescribed medications:

_____
_____
_____

What I can expect before my next prenatal visit:

_____
_____
_____

Instructions from my doctor:

_____
_____
_____

How much weight I should gain:

_____
_____
_____

Notes:

_____
_____
_____
_____
_____

My Prenatal Visits

Visit #9

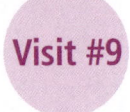

Prenatal provider seen:

Date:

The week of my pregnancy:

Weight:

Weight gain since the start of my pregnancy:

Blood pressure:

Fundal height:

Baby's heart rate:

Other tests:

Prescribed medications:

What I can expect before my next prenatal visit:

Instructions from my doctor:

How much weight I should gain:

Notes:

My Prenatal Visits

Visit #10

Prenatal provider seen:

Date:

The week of my pregnancy:

Weight:

Weight gain since the start of my pregnancy:

Blood pressure:

Fundal height:

Baby's heart rate:

Other tests:

Prescribed medications:

What I can expect before my next prenatal visit:

Instructions from my doctor:

How much weight I should gain:

Notes:

My Prenatal Visits

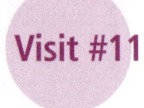

Visit #11

Prenatal provider seen:

Date:

The week of my pregnancy:

Weight:

Weight gain since the start of my pregnancy:

Blood pressure:

Fundal height:

Baby's heart rate:

Other tests:

Prescribed medications:

What I can expect before my next prenatal visit:

Instructions from my doctor:

How much weight I should gain:

Notes:

My Prenatal Visits

Visit #12

Prenatal provider seen:

Date:

The week of my pregnancy:

Weight:

Weight gain since the start of my pregnancy:

Blood pressure:

Fundal height:

Baby's heart rate:

Other tests:

Prescribed medications:

What I can expect before my next prenatal visit:

Instructions from my doctor:

How much weight I should gain:

Notes:

Monitoring My Baby's Movements

It will likely sink in that you're really, truly pregnant when you first feel your baby move, which typically happens around 20 weeks. As your baby grows, you may be concerned if you notice a reduction in your baby's activity rate. If so, you can count kicks. Here's how:

1. After eating a meal or snack, sit or lie down comfortably in a quiet place with no distractions.

2. Write down the time; then count the first 10 movements (kicks or elbows) you feel. Don't count hiccups. It should take your baby no longer than 1 hour to move 10 times.

3. Write down your baby's kick rate and then count again the next day at about the same time. Your baby should be moving about the same amount each day.

4. If your baby's activity level drops dramatically, call your doctor. It may be that your baby simply isn't feeling well or is less active, but it's worth checking with your provider.

Kick count: _____

Date: _____

Time: _____

How long it took to feel 10 kicks: _____

_____

_____

Kick count: _____

Date: _____

Time: _____

How long it took to feel 10 kicks: _____

_____

_____

Kick count:

Date:

Time:

How long it took to feel 10 kicks:

Kick count:

Date:

Time:

How long it took to feel 10 kicks:

Kick count:

Date:

Time:

How long it took to feel 10 kicks:

Kick count:

Date:

Time:

How long it took to feel 10 kicks:

Monitoring My Baby's Movements

Kick count:

Date:

Time:

How long it took to feel 10 kicks:

Kick count:

Date:

Time:

How long it took to feel 10 kicks:

Kick count:

Date:

Time:

How long it took to feel 10 kicks:

Kick count:

Date:

Time:

How long it took to feel 10 kicks:

Kick count:

Date:

Time:

How long it took to feel 10 kicks:

Kick count:

Date:

Time:

How long it took to feel 10 kicks:

Kick count:

Date:

Time:

How long it took to feel 10 kicks:

Kick count:

Date:

Time:

How long it took to feel 10 kicks:

Finding a Pediatrician

It's best to begin looking for a pediatrician long before your baby arrives. Start by asking friends for recommendations. Then call the doctors' offices and ask for a meet-and-greet appointment or phone interview. Here are some questions to ask the office staff or the doctor.

Interview #1

Pediatrician's name:

Office address:

Phone number:

Office hours:

SUGGESTED QUESTIONS:

Do you have weekend appointments?

How are middle-of-the-night emergencies handled?

Are same-day appointments available when my child gets sick?

Is my health insurance accepted by your practice? If so, does the office bill my insurance company, or do I have to pay up front and be reimbursed?
_____
_____
_____

Is there someone on staff who can help me with breastfeeding issues?
_____
_____
_____

To what hospitals do you admit patients?
_____
_____
_____

Other questions:
_____
_____
_____

Interview #2

Pediatrician's name: _____

Office address: _____
_____

Phone number: _____

Office hours: _____

SUGGESTED QUESTIONS:

Do you have weekend appointments?
_____
_____

Finding a Pediatrician

How are middle-of-the-night emergencies handled?

Are same-day appointments available when my child gets sick?

Is my health insurance accepted by your practice? If so, does the office bill my insurance company, or do I have to pay up front and be reimbursed?

Is there someone on staff who can help me with breastfeeding issues?

To what hospitals do you admit patients?

Other questions:

My Firsts

Record these important milestones, along with your emotions at the time. They'll make terrific entries in your little one's baby book.

First time **I heard my baby's heartbeat:**
_____
_____
_____

First time **I felt my baby kick:**
_____
_____
_____

First time **I felt my baby hiccup:**
_____
_____
_____

First time **I could no longer see my feet:**
_____
_____
_____

First time **I saw my baby on an ultrasound:**
_____
_____
_____

First time **my parents found out I was having this baby:**
_____
_____
_____

My Firsts

First time **I couldn't button my pants:**

First time **I wore a maternity dress:**

First time **I bought a new-baby outfit:**

First time **I experienced morning sickness:**

First time **a stranger asked me if I was pregnant:**

First time **it really sank in that I was going to be a mom:**

Eat, Drink (Water), and Be Merry

2

My Food and Diet Progress 86
My Food Cravings .128

Eat, Drink (Water), and Be Merry

2

A healthful diet and regular exercise are critical components of a healthy, happy pregnancy—and a healthy, happy baby. While getting all the nutrients your body needs is crucial, it's also important to indulge your cravings every once in a while, even if they're for double-chocolate chip ice cream. Use this handy section to ensure you're staying on track (at least most of the time).

My Food and Diet Progress

Use this 42-week chart to log whether you've taken your prenatal vitamins, done enough exercise, drunk sufficient fluids, and eaten the recommended servings of all the important foods.

Week #1

Date: _____

	S	M	T	W	Th	F	S
Prenatal vitamins							
Exercise (number of minutes)							
Fluids (number of 8-oz glasses)							
Prescribed medications: _____							
_____							
Fruits (3–4 servings/day)							
Vegetables (3–5 servings/day)							
Dairy foods (3 servings/day)							
Whole grains (3–6 servings/day)							
Protein (2–3 servings/day)							

Notes on how I'm feeling this week:

_____
_____
_____
_____
_____
_____

Week #2

Date: _____

	S	M	T	W	Th	F	S
Prenatal vitamins							
Exercise (number of minutes)							
Fluids (number of 8-oz glasses)							
Prescribed medications: _____							
_____							
Fruits (3–4 servings/day)							
Vegetables (3–5 servings/day)							
Dairy foods (3 servings/day)							
Whole grains (3–6 servings/day)							
Protein (2–3 servings/day)							

Notes on how I'm feeling this week:

_____

_____

_____

> **motherly ADVICE**
>
> **Yes, there can be too much of a good thing.** Never take more vitamins than your doctor tells you to. Megadoses of certain vitamins and minerals can harm your baby.

My Food and Diet Progress

Week #3

Date: _____

	S	M	T	W	Th	F	S
Prenatal vitamins							
Exercise (number of minutes)							
Fluids (number of 8-oz glasses)							
Prescribed medications: _____ _____							
Fruits (3–4 servings/day)							
Vegetables (3–5 servings/day)							
Dairy foods (3 servings/day)							
Whole grains (3–6 servings/day)							
Protein (2–3 servings/day)							

Notes on how I'm feeling this week:

_____
_____
_____
_____
_____
_____
_____

My Food and Diet Progress

Week #4

Date: _____

	S	M	T	W	Th	F	S
Prenatal vitamins							
Exercise (number of minutes)							
Fluids (number of 8-oz glasses)							
Prescribed medications: _____ _____							
Fruits (3–4 servings/day)							
Vegetables (3–5 servings/day)							
Dairy foods (3 servings/day)							
Whole grains (3–6 servings/day)							
Protein (2–3 servings/day)							

Notes on how I'm feeling this week:

_____
_____
_____
_____
_____
_____
_____

My Food and Diet Progress

Week #5

Date:_____

	S	M	T	W	Th	F	S
Prenatal vitamins							
Exercise (number of minutes)							
Fluids (number of 8-oz glasses)							
Prescribed medications: _____							
_____							
Fruits (3–4 servings/day)							
Vegetables (3–5 servings/day)							
Dairy foods (3 servings/day)							
Whole grains (3–6 servings/day)							
Protein (2–3 servings/day)							

Notes on how I'm feeling this week:

_____
_____
_____
_____
_____
_____
_____

My Food and Diet Progress

Week #6

Date: _____

	S	M	T	W	Th	F	S
Prenatal vitamins							
Exercise (number of minutes)							
Fluids (number of 8-oz glasses)							
Prescribed medications: _____							
_____							
Fruits (3–4 servings/day)							
Vegetables (3–5 servings/day)							
Dairy foods (3 servings/day)							
Whole grains (3–6 servings/day)							
Protein (2–3 servings/day)							

Notes on how I'm feeling this week:

My Food and Diet Progress

Week #7

Date:_____

	S	M	T	W	Th	F	S
Prenatal vitamins							
Exercise (number of minutes)							
Fluids (number of 8-oz glasses)							
Prescribed medications: _____ _____							
Fruits (3–4 servings/day)							
Vegetables (3–5 servings/day)							
Dairy foods (3 servings/day)							
Whole grains (3–6 servings/day)							
Protein (2–3 servings/day)							

Notes on how I'm feeling this week:

_____
_____
_____
_____
_____
_____
_____

Week #8

Date: _____

	S	M	T	W	Th	F	S
Prenatal vitamins							
Exercise (number of minutes)							
Fluids (number of 8-oz glasses)							
Prescribed medications: _____ _____							
Fruits (3–4 servings/day)							
Vegetables (3–5 servings/day)							
Dairy foods (3 servings/day)							
Whole grains (3–6 servings/day)							
Protein (2–3 servings/day)							

Notes on how I'm feeling this week:

_____
_____
_____
_____
_____
_____
_____

My Food and Diet Progress

Week #9

Date: _____

	S	M	T	W	Th	F	S

Prenatal vitamins

Exercise
(number of minutes)

Fluids
(number of 8-oz glasses)

Prescribed medications:

_____

_____

Fruits
(3–4 servings/day)

Vegetables
(3–5 servings/day)

Dairy foods
(3 servings/day)

Whole grains
(3–6 servings/day)

Protein
(2–3 servings/day)

Notes on how I'm feeling this week:

_____

_____

_____

_____

_____

_____

_____

Week #10

Date: _____

	S	M	T	W	Th	F	S
Prenatal vitamins							
Exercise (number of minutes)							
Fluids (number of 8-oz glasses)							
Prescribed medications: _____							
_____							
Fruits (3–4 servings/day)							
Vegetables (3–5 servings/day)							
Dairy foods (3 servings/day)							
Whole grains (3–6 servings/day)							
Protein (2–3 servings/day)							

Notes on how I'm feeling this week: _____

_____

_____

_____

_____

_____

_____

My Food and Diet Progress

Week #11

Date: _____

	S	M	T	W	Th	F	S
Prenatal vitamins							
Exercise (number of minutes)							
Fluids (number of 8-oz glasses)							
Prescribed medications: _____ _____							
Fruits (3–4 servings/day)							
Vegetables (3–5 servings/day)							
Dairy foods (3 servings/day)							
Whole grains (3–6 servings/day)							
Protein (2–3 servings/day)							

Notes on how I'm feeling this week:

_____
_____
_____
_____
_____
_____
_____
_____

Week #12

Date: _____

	S	M	T	W	Th	F	S
Prenatal vitamins							
Exercise (number of minutes)							
Fluids (number of 8-oz glasses)							
Prescribed medications: _____ _____							
Fruits (3–4 servings/day)							
Vegetables (3–5 servings/day)							
Dairy foods (3 servings/day)							
Whole grains (3–6 servings/day)							
Protein (2–3 servings/day)							

Notes on how I'm feeling this week:

_____
_____
_____

motherly ADVICE **You've likely figured out by now** that nausea can strike anytime, anywhere. Be prepared with an emergency kit that includes plastic bags, wet wipes, napkins, water for rinsing your mouth, a toothbrush and toothpaste, and breath mints.

My Food and Diet Progress

Week #13

Date:_____

	S	M	T	W	Th	F	S
Prenatal vitamins							
Exercise (number of minutes)							
Fluids (number of 8-oz glasses)							
Prescribed medications: _____							
Fruits (3–4 servings/day)							
Vegetables (3–5 servings/day)							
Dairy foods (3 servings/day)							
Whole grains (3–6 servings/day)							
Protein (2–3 servings/day)							

Notes on how I'm feeling this week: _____

_____

_____

_____

_____

_____

_____

Week #14

Date: _____

	S	M	T	W	Th	F	S
Prenatal vitamins							
Exercise (number of minutes)							
Fluids (number of 8-oz glasses)							
Prescribed medications: _____ _____							
Fruits (3–4 servings/day)							
Vegetables (3–5 servings/day)							
Dairy foods (3 servings/day)							
Whole grains (3–6 servings/day)							
Protein (2–3 servings/day)							

Notes on how I'm feeling this week:

_____
_____
_____
_____
_____
_____
_____

My Food and Diet Progress

Week #15

Date: _____

	S	M	T	W	Th	F	S
Prenatal vitamins							
Exercise (number of minutes)							
Fluids (number of 8-oz glasses)							
Prescribed medications: _____							
Fruits (3–4 servings/day)							
Vegetables (3–5 servings/day)							
Dairy foods (3 servings/day)							
Whole grains (3–6 servings/day)							
Protein (2–3 servings/day)							

Notes on how I'm feeling this week:

_____

_____

_____

_____

_____

_____

Week #16

Date: _____

	S	M	T	W	Th	F	S

Prenatal vitamins

Exercise
(number of minutes)

Fluids
(number of 8-oz glasses)

Prescribed medications:
_____
_____

Fruits
(3–4 servings/day)

Vegetables
(3–5 servings/day)

Dairy foods
(3 servings/day)

Whole grains
(3–6 servings/day)

Protein
(2–3 servings/day)

Notes on how I'm feeling this week:
_____
_____
_____
_____
_____
_____
_____

My Food and Diet Progress

Week #17

Date:_____

	S	M	T	W	Th	F	S
Prenatal vitamins							
Exercise (number of minutes)							
Fluids (number of 8-oz glasses)							
Prescribed medications: _____ _____							
Fruits (3–4 servings/day)							
Vegetables (3–5 servings/day)							
Dairy foods (3 servings/day)							
Whole grains (3–6 servings/day)							
Protein (2–3 servings/day)							

Notes on how I'm feeling this week:
_____
_____
_____
_____
_____
_____
_____
_____

Week #18

Date: _____

	S	M	T	W	Th	F	S
Prenatal vitamins							
Exercise (number of minutes)							
Fluids (number of 8-oz glasses)							
Prescribed medications: _____ _____							
Fruits (3–4 servings/day)							
Vegetables (3–5 servings/day)							
Dairy foods (3 servings/day)							
Whole grains (3–6 servings/day)							
Protein (2–3 servings/day)							

Notes on how I'm feeling this week:

_____

_____

_____

_____

_____

_____

_____

My Food and Diet Progress

Week #19

Date:_____

	S	M	T	W	Th	F	S
Prenatal vitamins							
Exercise (number of minutes)							
Fluids (number of 8-oz glasses)							
Prescribed medications: _____ _____							
Fruits (3–4 servings/day)							
Vegetables (3–5 servings/day)							
Dairy foods (3 servings/day)							
Whole grains (3–6 servings/day)							
Protein (2–3 servings/day)							

Notes on how I'm feeling this week:
_____
_____
_____

> **doctor's ADVICE**
>
> **If you haven't started taking prenatal vitamins yet** (some women start before they conceive), start taking them today—and take them every day without fail. Prenatal vitamins contain folic acid, which reduces the risk of birth defects. You can buy over-the-counter prenatal vitamins at most drugstores; ask the pharmacist if you have any questions.

Week #20

Date: _____

	S	M	T	W	Th	F	S
Prenatal vitamins							
Exercise (number of minutes)							
Fluids (number of 8-oz glasses)							
Prescribed medications: _____ _____							
Fruits (3–4 servings/day)							
Vegetables (3–5 servings/day)							
Dairy foods (3 servings/day)							
Whole grains (3–6 servings/day)							
Protein (2–3 servings/day)							

Notes on how I'm feeling this week:

_____
_____
_____
_____
_____
_____
_____

My Food and Diet Progress

Week #21

Date:_____

	S	M	T	W	Th	F	S
Prenatal vitamins							
Exercise (number of minutes)							
Fluids (number of 8-oz glasses)							
Prescribed medications: _____ _____							
Fruits (3–4 servings/day)							
Vegetables (3–5 servings/day)							
Dairy foods (3 servings/day)							
Whole grains (3–6 servings/day)							
Protein (2–3 servings/day)							

Notes on how I'm feeling this week:

_____
_____
_____
_____
_____
_____
_____

Week #21

Date: _____

	S	M	T	W	Th	F	S
Prenatal vitamins							
Exercise (number of minutes)							
Fluids (number of 8-oz glasses)							
Prescribed medications: _____ _____							
Fruits (3–4 servings/day)							
Vegetables (3–5 servings/day)							
Dairy foods (3 servings/day)							
Whole grains (3–6 servings/day)							
Protein (2–3 servings/day)							

Notes on how I'm feeling this week:

_____
_____
_____
_____
_____
_____
_____

My Food and Diet Progress

Week #23

Date:_____

	S	M	T	W	Th	F	S

Prenatal vitamins

Exercise
(number of minutes)

Fluids
(number of 8-oz glasses)

Prescribed medications:

_____

_____

Fruits
(3–4 servings/day)

Vegetables
(3–5 servings/day)

Dairy foods
(3 servings/day)

Whole grains
(3–6 servings/day)

Protein
(2–3 servings/day)

Notes on how I'm feeling this week:

_____

_____

_____

_____

_____

_____

_____

Week #24

Date: _____

	S	M	T	W	Th	F	S

Prenatal vitamins

Exercise
(number of minutes)

Fluids
(number of 8-oz glasses)

Prescribed medications:

_____

_____

Fruits
(3–4 servings/day)

Vegetables
(3–5 servings/day)

Dairy foods
(3 servings/day)

Whole grains
(3–6 servings/day)

Protein
(2–3 servings/day)

Notes on how I'm feeling this week:

_____

_____

_____

motherly ADVICE Because most fish contains some mercury, which can harm a baby's developing nervous system, pregnant women should not eat certain types of fish and shellfish and should limit their consumption of other types. For more information, visit the Environmental Protection Agency (EPA) website at www.epa.gov/ost/fish.

My Food and Diet Progress

Week #25

Date:_____

	S	M	T	W	Th	F	S
Prenatal vitamins							
Exercise (number of minutes)							
Fluids (number of 8-oz glasses)							
Prescribed medications: _____ _____							
Fruits (3–4 servings/day)							
Vegetables (3–5 servings/day)							
Dairy foods (3 servings/day)							
Whole grains (3–6 servings/day)							
Protein (2–3 servings/day)							

Notes on how I'm feeling this week:
_____
_____
_____
_____
_____
_____
_____
_____

Week #26

Date: _____

	S	M	T	W	Th	F	S
Prenatal vitamins							
Exercise (number of minutes)							
Fluids (number of 8-oz glasses)							
Prescribed medications: _____ _____							
Fruits (3–4 servings/day)							
Vegetables (3–5 servings/day)							
Dairy foods (3 servings/day)							
Whole grains (3–6 servings/day)							
Protein (2–3 servings/day)							

Notes on how I'm feeling this week:

_____
_____
_____
_____
_____
_____
_____

My Food and Diet Progress

Week #27

Date:_____

	S	M	T	W	Th	F	S
Prenatal vitamins							
Exercise (number of minutes)							
Fluids (number of 8-oz glasses)							
Prescribed medications: _____							
_____							
Fruits (3–4 servings/day)							
Vegetables (3–5 servings/day)							
Dairy foods (3 servings/day)							
Whole grains (3–6 servings/day)							
Protein (2–3 servings/day)							

Notes on how I'm feeling this week:

_____
_____
_____
_____
_____
_____
_____

Week #28

Date: _____

	S	M	T	W	Th	F	S
Prenatal vitamins							
Exercise (number of minutes)							
Fluids (number of 8-oz glasses)							
Prescribed medications: _____ _____							
Fruits (3–4 servings/day)							
Vegetables (3–5 servings/day)							
Dairy foods (3 servings/day)							
Whole grains (3–6 servings/day)							
Protein (2–3 servings/day)							

Notes on how I'm feeling this week:

_____

_____

_____

_____

_____

_____

_____

My Food and Diet Progress

Week #29

Date: _____

	S	M	T	W	Th	F	S
Prenatal vitamins							
Exercise (number of minutes)							
Fluids (number of 8-oz glasses)							
Prescribed medications: _____							
_____							
Fruits (3–4 servings/day)							
Vegetables (3–5 servings/day)							
Dairy foods (3 servings/day)							
Whole grains (3–6 servings/day)							
Protein (2–3 servings/day)							

Notes on how I'm feeling this week:

_____
_____
_____
_____
_____
_____
_____
_____

Week #30

Date: _____

	S	M	T	W	Th	F	S
Prenatal vitamins							
Exercise (number of minutes)							
Fluids (number of 8-oz glasses)							
Prescribed medications: _____ _____							
Fruits (3–4 servings/day)							
Vegetables (3–5 servings/day)							
Dairy foods (3 servings/day)							
Whole grains (3–6 servings/day)							
Protein (2–3 servings/day)							

Notes on how I'm feeling this week:

_____
_____
_____
_____
_____
_____
_____

My Food and Diet Progress

Week #31

Date: _____

	S	M	T	W	Th	F	S
Prenatal vitamins							
Exercise (number of minutes)							
Fluids (number of 8-oz glasses)							
Prescribed medications: _____ _____							
Fruits (3–4 servings/day)							
Vegetables (3–5 servings/day)							
Dairy foods (3 servings/day)							
Whole grains (3–6 servings/day)							
Protein (2–3 servings/day)							

Notes on how I'm feeling this week:

_____
_____
_____
_____
_____
_____
_____

Week #32

Date:_____

	S	M	T	W	Th	F	S
Prenatal vitamins							
Exercise (number of minutes)							
Fluids (number of 8-oz glasses)							
Prescribed medications: _____							
_____							
Fruits (3–4 servings/day)							
Vegetables (3–5 servings/day)							
Dairy foods (3 servings/day)							
Whole grains (3–6 servings/day)							
Protein (2–3 servings/day)							

Notes on how I'm feeling this week:

_____
_____
_____
_____
_____
_____
_____
_____

My Food and Diet Progress

Week #33

Date: _____

	S	M	T	W	Th	F	S
Prenatal vitamins							
Exercise (number of minutes)							
Fluids (number of 8-oz glasses)							
Prescribed medications: _____ _____							
Fruits (3–4 servings/day)							
Vegetables (3–5 servings/day)							
Dairy foods (3 servings/day)							
Whole grains (3–6 servings/day)							
Protein (2–3 servings/day)							

Notes on how I'm feeling this week: _____

_____

---

motherly ADVICE

Bored with drinking the recommended 8 glasses of water a day? Consider these alternatives: Drink milk, decaffeinated tea or coffee, fruit juice, seltzer, or sports drinks; suck on ice chips; or eat frozen juice bars and water-filled fruits such as watermelon and grapes.

Week #34

Date: _____

	S	M	T	W	Th	F	S
Prenatal vitamins							
Exercise (number of minutes)							
Fluids (number of 8-oz glasses)							
Prescribed medications: _____							
_____							
Fruits (3–4 servings/day)							
Vegetables (3–5 servings/day)							
Dairy foods (3 servings/day)							
Whole grains (3–6 servings/day)							
Protein (2–3 servings/day)							

Notes on how I'm feeling this week:

_____
_____
_____
_____
_____
_____
_____

My Food and Diet Progress

Week #35

Date: _____

	S	M	T	W	Th	F	S

Prenatal vitamins

Exercise
(number of minutes)

Fluids
(number of 8-oz glasses)

Prescribed medications:
_____

_____

Fruits
(3–4 servings/day)

Vegetables
(3–5 servings/day)

Dairy foods
(3 servings/day)

Whole grains
(3–6 servings/day)

Protein
(2–3 servings/day)

Notes on how I'm feeling this week:

_____

_____

_____

_____

_____

_____

_____

Week #36

Date: _____

	S	M	T	W	Th	F	S
Prenatal vitamins							
Exercise (number of minutes)							
Fluids (number of 8-oz glasses)							
Prescribed medications: _____ _____							
Fruits (3–4 servings/day)							
Vegetables (3–5 servings/day)							
Dairy foods (3 servings/day)							
Whole grains (3–6 servings/day)							
Protein (2–3 servings/day)							

Notes on how I'm feeling this week:

_____
_____
_____
_____
_____
_____
_____

My Food and Diet Progress

Week #37

Date: _____

	S	M	T	W	Th	F	S
Prenatal vitamins							
Exercise (number of minutes)							
Fluids (number of 8-oz glasses)							
Prescribed medications: _____ _____							
Fruits (3–4 servings/day)							
Vegetables (3–5 servings/day)							
Dairy foods (3 servings/day)							
Whole grains (3–6 servings/day)							
Protein (2–3 servings/day)							

Notes on how I'm feeling this week:

_____
_____
_____
_____
_____
_____
_____

My Food and Diet Progress

Week #38

Date: _____

	S	M	T	W	Th	F	S
Prenatal vitamins							
Exercise (number of minutes)							
Fluids (number of 8-oz glasses)							
Prescribed medications: _____ _____							
Fruits (3–4 servings/day)							
Vegetables (3–5 servings/day)							
Dairy foods (3 servings/day)							
Whole grains (3–6 servings/day)							
Protein (2–3 servings/day)							

Notes on how I'm feeling this week:

_____
_____
_____
_____
_____
_____
_____

My Food and Diet Progress

Week #39

Date: _____

Prenatal vitamins

Exercise
(number of minutes)

Fluids
(number of 8-oz glasses)

Prescribed medications:
_____
_____

Fruits
(3–4 servings/day)

Vegetables
(3–5 servings/day)

Dairy foods
(3 servings/day)

Whole grains
(3–6 servings/day)

Protein
(2–3 servings/day)

Notes on how I'm feeling this week:
_____
_____
_____
_____
_____
_____
_____

Week #40

Date: _____

	S	M	T	W	Th	F	S
Prenatal vitamins							
Exercise (number of minutes)							
Fluids (number of 8-oz glasses)							
Prescribed medications: _____ _____							
Fruits (3–4 servings/day)							
Vegetables (3–5 servings/day)							
Dairy foods (3 servings/day)							
Whole grains (3–6 servings/day)							
Protein (2–3 servings/day)							

Notes on how I'm feeling this week:

---

doctor's ADVICE

You're at 40 weeks—so why hasn't your baby made his big arrival yet? The truth is that 80 percent of babies arrive between 38 weeks and 42 weeks of pregnancy, so you may have a couple of weeks still to go.

My Food and Diet Progress

Week #41

Date: _____

	S	M	T	W	Th	F	S
Prenatal vitamins							
Exercise (number of minutes)							
Fluids (number of 8-oz glasses)							
Prescribed medications: _____ _____							
Fruits (3–4 servings/day)							
Vegetables (3–5 servings/day)							
Dairy foods (3 servings/day)							
Whole grains (3–6 servings/day)							
Protein (2–3 servings/day)							

Notes on how I'm feeling this week:

_____
_____
_____
_____
_____
_____
_____

Week #42

Date: _____

	S	M	T	W	Th	F	S
Prenatal vitamins							
Exercise (number of minutes)							
Fluids (number of 8-oz glasses)							
Prescribed medications: _____							
_____							
Fruits (3–4 servings/day)							
Vegetables (3–5 servings/day)							
Dairy foods (3 servings/day)							
Whole grains (3–6 servings/day)							
Protein (2–3 servings/day)							

Notes on how I'm feeling this week:

_____

_____

_____

motherly ADVICE **Food poisoning affects 76 million Americans a year,** and pregnant women are among the most vulnerable. Protect yourself by washing your hands throughout the day and before and after preparing foods; avoid eating foods that contain raw eggs; wash fruits and vegetables thoroughly; and throw away any food that's been sitting out on a counter for more than 2 hours.

My Food Cravings

Are you a pickle-and-ice-cream fanatic? Or is your fridge filled with peanut butter? Jot down your unusual cravings and when you had them. In a few years, look back and see if what you ate relates to what your child likes to eat.

What I craved: **During Week #:**

Notes:

What I craved: **During Week #:**

Notes:

What I craved: **During Week #:**

Notes:

What I craved: **During Week #:**

Notes:

What I craved: **During Week #:**

Notes:

What I craved: **During Week #:**

Notes:

What I craved: _____ **During Week #:** _____

Notes: _____

_____

What I craved: _____ **During Week #:** _____

Notes: _____

_____

What I craved: _____ **During Week #:** _____

Notes: _____

_____

What I craved: _____ **During Week #:** _____

Notes: _____

_____

What I craved: _____ **During Week #:** _____

Notes: _____

_____

What I craved: _____ **During Week #:** _____

Notes: _____

_____

What I craved: _____ **During Week #:** _____

Notes: _____

My Food Cravings

What I craved: _____ **During Week #:** _____

Notes: _____

_____

What I craved: _____ **During Week #:** _____

Notes: _____

_____

What I craved: _____ **During Week #:** _____

Notes: _____

_____

What I craved: _____ **During Week #:** _____

Notes: _____

_____

What I craved: _____ **During Week #:** _____

Notes: _____

_____

What I craved: _____ **During Week #:** _____

Notes: _____

_____

What I craved: _____ **During Week #:** _____

Notes: _____

At Work and at Home

3

Evaluating Home Hazards 132

Evaluating Work Hazards 136

Maternity Leave 140

Final Checklist for Leaving Work 145

At Work and at Home

3

With a new baby on the way, it's time to take a fresh look at your home and your work environments. Conditions that are perfectly safe for an ordinary person can be hazardous for a pregnant woman or her baby. It takes only a few moments to make changes that will protect your baby, both before and after birth.

Evaluating Home Hazards

Are you exposed to environmental toxins at home? Do a survey of your living space using this checklist of possible dangers as a guide. Talk to your prenatal provider about any concerns you have.

Chemical insecticides Yes ☐ No ☐
(these may include sprays you use at home or larger-scale sprays, such as neighborhood-wide efforts by the city to control mosquitoes)

Dry-cleaning fluids Yes ☐ No ☐

Home cleaning products Yes ☐ No ☐

Oven cleaners Yes ☐ No ☐

Mold and mildew cleaners Yes ☐ No ☐

Lead in your tap water Yes ☐ No ☐
(check with your local Environmental Protection Agency about the quality of your home's tap water)

Lead paint Yes ☐ No ☐

Lead-lined pottery or china Yes ☐ No ☐
(most often found in dishes that are handmade or imported)

Oil-base paints Yes ☐ No ☐
(may contain dangerous solvents)

Paint removers Yes ☐ No ☐

Paint thinners Yes ☐ No ☐

My other concerns:

Evaluating Home Hazards

My other concerns:

Evaluating Work Hazards

What hazards at work could interfere with your baby's healthy development? Be on the lookout for these potential dangers. Talk to your provider about precautions you should take on the job.

Anesthetic gases	Yes ☐	No ☐
Benzene	Yes ☐	No ☐
Carbon monoxide	Yes ☐	No ☐
Chemotherapy drugs	Yes ☐	No ☐
Cleaning products	Yes ☐	No ☐
Ethylene oxide (used to sterilize medical equipment)	Yes ☐	No ☐
Formaldehyde	Yes ☐	No ☐
Glycol ethers (used in semiconductor plants)	Yes ☐	No ☐
Heavy lifting	Yes ☐	No ☐
Ionizing radiation	Yes ☐	No ☐
Lead	Yes ☐	No ☐
Lead paints	Yes ☐	No ☐
Mercury	Yes ☐	No ☐
Nitrous oxide	Yes ☐	No ☐
Organic solvents	Yes ☐	No ☐
Paint solvents	Yes ☐	No ☐
Paint thinners	Yes ☐	No ☐
Pesticides	Yes ☐	No ☐

Sitting for long periods	Yes ☐	No ☐
Standing for long periods	Yes ☐	No ☐
Stress (physical or emotional)	Yes ☐	No ☐
X-rays	Yes ☐	No ☐

My other concerns:

_____
_____
_____
_____
_____
_____
_____
_____

doctor's ADVICE

Ask your employer for the Material Safety Data Sheets for the products you use or contact the Occupational Safety and Health Administration (OSHA). For more information about the effect of workplace hazards on reproductive health and information on the federal laws that protect the health, safety, and employment rights of pregnant women at work, contact the National Institute for Occupational Safety and Health: (800) 356-4674 or www.cdc.gov/niosh.

Evaluating Work Hazards

My other concerns:

doctor's ADVICE **Most women with normal pregnancies** continue to work until very near their due dates. However, if you have a chronic illness such as diabetes or any pregnancy-induced conditions such as high blood pressure, you might have to cut back on your work hours or quit completely. You may also have to stop working sooner if you're carrying multiples or have any pregnancy history that could cause complications during your current pregnancy.

Maternity Leave

Take the time to plan carefully and prepare for your leave. Here are some questions to consider.

Ask your company's human resources manager:

☐ **What are the company's official benefits policies?**
_____
_____
_____

☐ **What am I entitled to by law?**
_____
_____
_____

☐ **Am I protected by the federal Family and Medical Leave Act (FMLA)?** (This law applies to all businesses with 50 or more employees.)
_____
_____
_____
_____

☐ **Can I continue to purchase health insurance through my company during and after maternity leave?**
_____
_____
_____

☐ Will my job—or a similar position—be available for me when I return from maternity leave?

☐ Does the company offer any paid maternity leave?

☐ For how many weeks?

☐ Does the company offer any unpaid maternity leave?

☐ For how many weeks?

☐ Can I borrow paid leave against future time off?

Maternity Leave

☐ **Can I use my vacation time?**

☐ **Can I use up my sick time?**

☐ **Are there any job-sharing opportunities available?**

☐ **Can I stagger my leave, taking a few weeks immediately after delivery and a few later? (If your partner will have paternity leave, this may make sense.)**

Consider what your long-term intentions are:

☐ **Do you want to return to work full-time?**
_____
_____
_____
_____

☐ **Do you want to return part-time?**
_____
_____
_____
_____

☐ **Do you want to quit and stop working entirely?**
_____
_____
_____
_____

☐ **Ideally, how long do you want to take for maternity leave?**
_____
_____
_____

☐ **When do you want to begin your maternity leave?**
_____

Maternity Leave

Other questions:

☐ How will my maternity leave affect my finances?
_____
_____
_____
_____

☐ Will my partner and I have to adjust our budget?
_____
_____
_____
_____

☐ Does my partner's employer offer paid or unpaid paternity leave?
_____
_____
_____
_____

☐ What arrangements have working mothers I know made with their companies?
_____
_____
_____
_____

Notes:
_____
_____

Final Checklist for Leaving Work

Before you head out of the office for the last time (or at least for a few weeks), get your desk in order. Whether you'll be returning to the job or not, it's always best to leave on a good note.

- [ ] Organize and clean up your desk.

- [ ] Remove any important personal belongings and photos.

- [ ] Set up a meeting with your replacement to smooth the transition. If that's not possible, leave detailed notes about your responsibilities.

- [ ] Return company-owned items such as laptop computers and cell phones, if necessary.

- [ ] Meet with your supervisor to go over your leave schedule and discuss last-minute items.

- [ ] Give your emergency contact information to a supervisor.

- [ ] Double-check that you've signed all necessary forms with human resources.

- [ ] Confirm that the payroll department knows where to send your paychecks.

- [ ] If you're not returning to your job, schedule an exit interview with your human resources department. Ask about transferring your pension benefits or 401(k) accounts into a personal account, how long your health insurance coverage will last, and so on.

- [ ] Thank your employer for the opportunities you've been given, especially if the company has been particularly accommodating with regard to your maternity leave requests.

Final Checklist for Leaving Work

Other reminders:

_____
_____
_____
_____
_____
_____
_____
_____
_____
_____
_____
_____
_____
_____
_____
_____
_____
_____

> **friendly ADVICE**
> **Congratulations, you have a new tax deduction!** If your baby will be born in the current tax year, adjust your tax withholding at work now to reflect your family's new addition.

And Baby Makes Three (or More!)

4

Go to the Head of the Class **148**
Retail Therapy **150**
Off to the Hospital **158**
Words of Wisdom **164**
It's Delivery Day! **166**
My Labor (Finally!) **168**
My Contractions **174**
My Labor and Delivery **177**
My Partner's Labor Experience **178**
My Labor Team **180**
Baby's First Visitors **182**
What a Surprise! **184**

# And Baby Makes Three (or More!)

4

Readying your household for the arrival of your little one is a joyful activity that requires lots of new gadgets, clothes, classes, and more. From decorating the nursery to buying a wardrobe of tiny baby clothes to wandering the aisles of the toy store, the preparations seem endless. Stay organized with this great section so you don't arrive home with items you've bought once (or twice) already.

Go to the Head of the Class

Classes offered by local hospitals and birth centers can be terrific for new parents-to-be or veteran parents who would like a refresher course in the basics. Look for topics such as childbirth, breastfeeding, baby care, planned cesarean deliveries, natural childbirth (giving birth without pain medication), and giving birth to multiples.

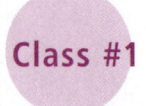

Class #1

TITLE/TOPIC:

Dates offered:

Times offered:

Fee:

Address:

Teacher's contact info:

Sign-up deadline:

Items to bring to class:

Class #2

TITLE/TOPIC:

Dates offered:

Times offered:

Fee:

Address:

Teacher's contact info:

Sign-up deadline:

Items to bring to class:

Retail Therapy: Baby Clothes

There's nothing like a shopping excursion for baby clothes and bottles to take your mind off your aching back. In fact, it's easy to get carried away and buy more than you need or will ever be able to use. These checklists will help keep your buying on track.

What you'll need

- [ ] 5–7 one-pieces
- [ ] 5–7 undershirts (short-sleeve or long-sleeve, depending on the season)
- [ ] 1 pair of cotton mittens (these protect babies from scratching themselves)
- [ ] 2 one-piece pajamas
- [ ] 5 pairs of socks
- [ ] 2–3 dress-up outfits
- [ ] Hats (for summer, choose one with a wide brim and a chin strap; for winter, choose something that's warm)
- [ ] A sweater, jacket, or fleece if the weather is cold (zip-up is easier to put on than over-the-head)
- [ ] A warm coat or baby bag that fits into the car seat
- [ ] Blankets

> **motherly ADVICE**
>
> **A new baby can strain a budget,** so borrow clothes, cribs, or strollers from parents who are no longer using the items. And ask up front if they'd like the items returned to them—or if you can pass the items along to another soon-to-be mom when you're finished.

My baby clothes wish list

DESCRIPTION	Have (number)	Will Buy (number)	Borrow (number)

Retail Therapy: Baby Care Supplies

What you'll need

- [ ] Diapers (disposable or cloth)
- [ ] Unscented wipes (disposable or cloth)
- [ ] Gentle baby soap
- [ ] No-tear shampoo
- [ ] Soft washcloths
- [ ] Baby nasal syringe
- [ ] Diaper cream
- [ ] Baby bathtub
- [ ] Baby nail clippers

> **motherly ADVICE** Oh, baby! Newborns can go through 10 to 12 diapers in a 24-hour period, so plan accordingly. If you're using disposables, buy enough to last a week or two, and you'll save yourself the aggravation of having to run to the store in the middle of the night. If you prefer cloth diapers, buy them a few weeks before your due date because new diapers should be washed several times before use.

Other items I need

DESCRIPTION	Have (number)	Will Buy (number)

Retail Therapy: Nursery Basics

What you'll need

- [ ] Crib
- [ ] Fitted crib sheets
- [ ] Padded bumpers for the crib
- [ ] Bassinet for newborns (optional)
- [ ] Changing table
- [ ] Changing pad with washable cover
- [ ] Rocking chair
- [ ] Garbage can with lid
- [ ] Laundry hamper
- [ ] Mobile for the crib
- [ ] Dimmer switch or three-way lamp for soft lighting
- [ ] White noise machine or CD player to help baby sleep

motherly ADVICE

The best time to take a childbirth class is during weeks 34–36. That way, you'll finish it about 4 weeks before you deliver—and the information will still be fresh when you head to the hospital.

My nursery wish list

DESCRIPTION	Have (number)	Will Buy (number)	Borrow (number)

Retail Therapy: Gear for Leaving the House

You certainly won't need all of these items; choose what makes sense for your situation.

What you'll need

- ☐ Diaper bag
- ☐ Stroller
- ☐ Jogger stroller
- ☐ Backpack
- ☐ Car seat
- ☐ Convertible frontpack/backpack
- ☐ Convertible stroller/backpack
- ☐ Sling

motherly ADVICE

In preparation for the little one, hang a whiteboard or chalkboard in the kitchen. Soon you'll use it to write notes to your partner (and visiting grandparents) to announce that you're out for a walk with the baby or that you need (more) diapers.

My gear wish list

DESCRIPTION	Have (number)	Will Buy (number)	Borrow (number)

Off to the Hospital

Reduce your stress by packing for your trip to the hospital a few weeks before your expected due date.

What Mom should pack

- [ ] Nightgown or long T-shirt for labor
- [ ] Robe
- [ ] Pajamas for sleeping
- [ ] Slippers
- [ ] Warm socks for the delivery room
- [ ] 5–6 pairs of underwear
- [ ] Hair products, such as a brush, hair dryer, and curling iron
- [ ] Toothpaste and toothbrush
- [ ] Travel-size shampoo and conditioner
- [ ] Soap
- [ ] Shower slippers
- [ ] A watch with a second hand for timing contractions
- [ ] Camera plus extra batteries
- [ ] Outfit to leave the hospital in (a maternity outfit is a good choice because you'll still have a fairly large belly)
- [ ] 2 nursing bras, if you're planning to breastfeed
- [ ] Lip balm
- [ ] Body lotion
- [ ] Several big, absorbent sanitary napkins
- [ ] CDs and CD player
- [ ] Magazines
- [ ] Tennis ball for labor massage
- [ ] Identification
- [ ] Insurance card

Other items I'd like to have with me

DESCRIPTION	Have (number)	Will Buy (number)	Borrow (number)

Off to the Hospital

What Dad should pack

- [ ] Deck of cards
- [ ] Bottled water
- [ ] Nonperishable snacks (granola bars, crackers, candy bars)
- [ ] Toothbrush, deodorant, and comb
- [ ] Razor
- [ ] Change for vending machines
- [ ] Change of clothes
- [ ] Soothing music to listen to during labor
- [ ] Portable music player
- [ ] Cell phone or calling card
- [ ] Name, address, and phone number of the hospital or birth center
- [ ] Contact information for your doctor or midwife and your doula, if you're using one
- [ ] Names and phone numbers of the people you've lined up to babysit your children, if you have other children
- [ ] Names and phone numbers of pet sitters, if you have pets
- [ ] Call list of relatives and friends
- [ ] Identification
- [ ] Insurance card

Other items to pack

☐ _____

☐ _____

☐ _____

☐ _____

☐ _____

☐ _____

☐ _____

☐ _____

☐ _____

☐ _____

☐ _____

motherly ADVICE **If you'd like champagne or sparkling cider** to make a toast to your new baby, buy it now and write your name in marker on the label so it doesn't get misplaced at the hospital or birth center.

Off to the Hospital

What to pack for baby

- [ ] 3–4 undershirts and one-pieces
- [ ] A special outfit and cap to wear home
- [ ] Receiving blanket
- [ ] Warm coat and hat, if it's cold
- [ ] Camera or video recorder for documenting baby's first days of life

Other items I'd like to bring

- [ ] _____
- [ ] _____
- [ ] _____
- [ ] _____
- [ ] _____

> **motherly ADVICE** **Install your baby's infant car seat** in the backseat of your car a week or two before your due date. Getting the seat in correctly can be tricky, so drive your car to a free child safety seat inspection station. Visit the Safe Kids Worldwide website at www.safekids.org to find one near you.

Other items I'd like to bring

☐ _____

☐ _____

☐ _____

☐ _____

☐ _____

☐ _____

☐ _____

☐ _____

☐ _____

☐ _____

☐ _____

☐ _____

☐ _____

Words of Wisdom

Once you're pregnant, it will seem as if every mom you talk to gives you advice, whether it's about handling morning sickness or surviving labor pains. Write down the good, the bad, and the funny; then check back in a few months and see if any of it worked for you!

My friend's/family member's name:

Her advice:

My friend's/family member's name:

Her advice:

My friend's/family member's name:

Her advice:

_____
_____
_____
_____
_____
_____
_____
_____
_____
_____

My friend's/family member's name:

Her advice:

_____
_____
_____
_____
_____
_____
_____

It's Delivery Day!

When time is of the essence, call these important people:

HOSPITAL

Name:

Phone number:

Address:

PRENATAL PROVIDER

Name:

Phone number:

Address:

BABYSITTER

Name:

Phone number:

Address:

PET SITTER

Name:

Phone number:

Address:

TAXI COMPANY

Name: _____

Phone number: _____

Address: _____
_____
_____

YOUR EMPLOYER (IF YOU'RE STILL WORKING)

Name: _____

Phone number: _____

Address: _____
_____
_____

OTHERS

Name: _____

Phone number: _____

Address: _____
_____
_____

OTHERS

Name: _____

Phone number: _____

Address: _____

My Labor (Finally!)

My contractions started on (date/time):

At first they felt like:

They were this far apart:

They lasted this long:

The person I called first to tell:

His/her reaction:

My Labor (Finally!)

The person I called second:

His/her reaction:

What I was thinking:

I remembered these instructions from my doctor:

When I called my doctor:

What my doctor said:

My Labor (Finally!)

When my doctor told me to come to the hospital:

What I did at home while I waited to leave:

Who drove me to the hospital and when:

> **doctor's ADVICE**
> **When should you call your practitioner?** Follow the 1-5-1 rule: Pick up the phone when your contractions each last 1 minute or more, are no more than 5 minutes apart, and have been going on for 1 hour.

My Contractions

START TIME:

End time:

Length:

Time between contractions:

START TIME:

End time:

Length:

Time between contractions:

START TIME:

End time:

Length:

Time between contractions:

START TIME:

End time:

Length:

Time between contractions:

START TIME:

End time:

Length:

Time between contractions:

START TIME:

End time:

Length:

Time between contractions:

START TIME:

End time:

Length:

Time between contractions:

START TIME:

End time:

Length:

Time between contractions:

My Contractions

START TIME:

End time:

Length:

Time between contractions:

START TIME:

End time:

Length:

Time between contractions:

START TIME:

End time:

Length:

Time between contractions:

START TIME:

End time:

Length:

Time between contractions:

My Labor and Delivery

Date and time I was admitted to the hospital/birth center:

Date and time of my first exam:

When my water broke:

When I was fully dilated and started pushing:

Delivery date and time:

Baby's weight:

Baby's length:

Apgar scores:

My Partner's Labor Experience

Did your baby's father hold your hand during labor and delivery? Or was he so queasy that he had to spend the time in the waiting room? Ask your partner for his take on the events that occurred on delivery day.

My Labor Team

Some of your most important support—both physically and emotionally—has likely come from your expert labor team. Write down the names of these health care heroes and send them a note of appreciation.

MY NURSES:

MY DOCTOR OR MIDWIFE:

Baby's First Visitors

The first few hours of your baby's life will be filled with well-wishers bringing flowers, candy, and casseroles—and perhaps a few words of wisdom. Keep track of friends and family who made it to the hospital or who stopped by the house within a few days of your baby's arrival.

Who visited: _____

What was said: _____

_____

_____

_____

_____

Who visited: _____

What was said: _____

_____

_____

_____

_____

Who visited: _____

What was said: _____

_____

_____

_____

_____

Who visited: _____

What was said: _____

_____

_____

Who visited: _____
What was said: _____
_____
_____
_____

Who visited: _____
What was said: _____
_____
_____
_____

Who visited: _____
What was said: _____
_____
_____
_____

Who visited: _____
What was said: _____
_____
_____
_____

What a Surprise!

Whether this is your first pregnancy or your fourth, chances are you encountered a few surprises. After all, every pregnancy—like every baby—is unique. Were you shocked by how severe your morning sickness was? Surprised that you could still (barely) fit into your prepregnancy jeans at 5 months? Write down your observations.

It's a Celebration!

5

Baby Showers 186

Baby Announcements 192

Name Games 200

Phone or E-mail Tree 204

Handy Websites 207

It's a Celebration!

5

What a wonderful time this is! You'll soon be welcoming home a new addition to your family. Take a deep breath and savor these 9 months, which promise to be full of lots of surprises and love. Your life will soon be changed forever. When family and friends gather to share your good news, keep track of all the showers and celebrations and other festivities in this handy section. It'll be a great reminder of the good times and can serve as a mailing list for your thank-you notes!

Baby Showers

Choose a trusted friend (who has good penmanship!) to write down your gifts as you open them and ask her to note each gift giver's name. Remember to include gifts that get sent directly to your house.

DESCRIPTION OF GIFT	Who gave it	Thank-you note sent?
_____ _____ _____		Yes ☐

DESCRIPTION OF GIFT	Who gave it	Thank-you note sent?
_____ _____ _____		Yes ☐

DESCRIPTION OF GIFT	Who gave it	Thank-you note sent?
_____ _____ _____		Yes ☐

DESCRIPTION OF GIFT	Who gave it	Thank-you note sent?
_____ _____ _____		Yes ☐

DESCRIPTION OF GIFT	Who gave it	Thank-you note sent?
		Yes ☐
DESCRIPTION OF GIFT	Who gave it	Thank-you note sent?
		Yes ☐
DESCRIPTION OF GIFT	Who gave it	Thank-you note sent?
		Yes ☐
DESCRIPTION OF GIFT	Who gave it	Thank-you note sent?
		Yes ☐

Baby Showers

DESCRIPTION OF GIFT	Who gave it	Thank-you note sent?
		Yes ☐

DESCRIPTION OF GIFT	Who gave it	Thank-you note sent?
		Yes ☐

DESCRIPTION OF GIFT	Who gave it	Thank-you note sent?
		Yes ☐

DESCRIPTION OF GIFT	Who gave it	Thank-you note sent?
		Yes ☐

DESCRIPTION OF GIFT	Who gave it	Thank-you note sent?
_____ _____ _____		Yes ☐

DESCRIPTION OF GIFT	Who gave it	Thank-you note sent?
_____ _____ _____		Yes ☐

DESCRIPTION OF GIFT	Who gave it	Thank-you note sent?
_____ _____ _____		Yes ☐

DESCRIPTION OF GIFT	Who gave it	Thank-you note sent?
_____ _____ _____		Yes ☐

Baby Showers

DESCRIPTION OF GIFT	Who gave it	Thank-you note sent?
		Yes ☐

DESCRIPTION OF GIFT	Who gave it	Thank-you note sent?
		Yes ☐

DESCRIPTION OF GIFT	Who gave it	Thank-you note sent?
		Yes ☐

DESCRIPTION OF GIFT	Who gave it	Thank-you note sent?
		Yes ☐

DESCRIPTION OF GIFT	Who gave it	Thank-you note sent?
		Yes ☐
DESCRIPTION OF GIFT	Who gave it	Thank-you note sent?
		Yes ☐
DESCRIPTION OF GIFT	Who gave it	Thank-you note sent?
		Yes ☐
DESCRIPTION OF GIFT	Who gave it	Thank-you note sent?
		Yes ☐

Baby Announcements

Start spreading the news! Begin by listing the names and addresses of friends, relatives, and coworkers to whom you'd like to send baby announcements.

NAME:

Address:

E-mail address:

NAME:

Address:

E-mail address:

NAME:

Address:

E-mail address:

NAME:

Address:

E-mail address:

NAME:

Address:

E-mail address:

NAME:

Address:

E-mail address:

NAME:

Address:

E-mail address:

NAME:

Address:

E-mail address:

NAME:

Address:

E-mail address:

Baby Announcements

NAME:

Address:

E-mail address:

NAME:

Address:

E-mail address:

NAME:

Address:

E-mail address:

NAME:

Address:

E-mail address:

NAME:

Address:

E-mail address:

NAME:

Address:

E-mail address:

NAME:

Address:

E-mail address:

NAME:

Address:

E-mail address:

NAME:

Address:

E-mail address:

NAME:

Address:

E-mail address:

Baby Announcements

NAME:

Address:

E-mail address:

NAME:

Address:

E-mail address:

NAME:

Address:

E-mail address:

NAME:

Address:

E-mail address:

> **motherly ADVICE**
> **Address all your baby announcement** envelopes and add stamps before your due date so that you have one less thing to do once the new member of the family is born.

NAME:

Address:

E-mail address:

NAME:

Address:

E-mail address:

NAME:

Address:

E-mail address:

NAME:

Address:

E-mail address:

NAME:

Address:

E-mail address:

Baby Announcements

NAME:
_____

Address:
_____
_____

E-mail address:
_____

NAME:
_____

Address:
_____
_____

E-mail address:
_____

NAME:
_____

Address:
_____
_____

E-mail address:
_____

NAME:
_____

Address:
_____
_____

E-mail address:
_____

NAME:
_____

Address:
_____
_____

E-mail address:
_____

NAME:

Address:

E-mail address:

NAME:

Address:

E-mail address:

NAME:

Address:

E-mail address:

NAME:

Address:

E-mail address:

NAME:

Address:

E-mail address:

Name Games

Choosing a baby's name is a momentous decision for new parents. Are there any ethnic or religious traditions you or your partner would like to honor? Do you prefer traditional names? One-of-a-kind names? Names that start with a certain letter? Use these pages to keep track of names you and your partner like.

Names from your side of the family:

Name **Relation (grandparent, aunt, etc.)**

Names from your partner's side of the family:

Name   Relation (grandparent, aunt, etc.)

Name Games

Other names I like:

Name	Meaning

motherly ADVICE

To find out what names have been popular each year going back to the 1870s, check out the Social Security Administration's online name-tracking search engine at www.ssa.gov/OACT/babynames/. You'll also find information about getting your baby's own Social Security number.

Phone or E-mail Tree

As you talk to friends and relatives over the months, jot down their contact information here; then use it to prepare a "phone tree" or a mass e-mail message that can be sent out within hours of your new baby's arrival.

NAME:

Phone number:

E-mail address:

NAME:

Phone number:

E-mail address:

NAME:

Phone number:

E-mail address:

NAME:

Phone number:

E-mail address:

NAME:

Phone number:

E-mail address:

NAME:

Phone number:

E-mail address:

NAME:

Phone number:

E-mail address:

NAME:

Phone number:

E-mail address:

NAME

Phone number:

E-mail address:

Phone or E-mail Tree

NAME:

Phone number:

E-mail address:

NAME:

Phone number:

E-mail address:

NAME:

Phone number:

E-mail address:

NAME:

Phone number:

E-mail address:

motherly ADVICE **Does your hospital or birth center post new babies'** pictures on its website? If so, get the website address so you can share one of baby's first photos with friends and family.

Handy Websites

These are some of the great websites recommended in this book. Log on and get informed!

www.cdc.gov/niosh: National Institute for Occupational Safety and Health

www.ssa.gov/OACT/babynames/: Social Security Administration's online name-tracking search engine

www.epa.gov/ost/fish: Environmental Protection Agency's fish advisories

www.safekids.org: Safe Kids Worldwide

Other informational sites:

www.marchofdimes.com: March of Dimes

www.eatright.org: American Dietetic Association

www.midwife.org: American College of Nurse-Midwives

Other good websites I like to visit:

_____
_____
_____
_____
_____
_____
_____
_____
_____
_____

You & Your BABY™
Essential Books
for Life's Most Amazing Journey

You & Your Baby: Pregnancy
Up-to-date, comprehensive pregnancy guide containing straightforward, comforting, expert advice that explains, week-by-week, everything expectant parents need to know about pregnancy and birth. Includes amazing full-color in-utero fetal photos that deliver an unforgettable visual journey of developing life.

You & Your Baby: Pregnancy Organizer
Ideal companion for mother-to-be, helping them to track and prepare for important events such as prenatal appointments, questions for the doctor, medications, diet plans, and more. Includes helpful checklists, shopping wish lists, and places to record memorable milestones such as baby's first kick.

All new *You & Your Baby* pregnancy book series authored by nationally recognized physician, Dr. Laura Riley.

Found wherever Pregnancy and Childbirth books are sold.